The New Atkins Diet Quick Start Guide

The New Atkins Diet Quick Start Guide

A Faster, Simpler Way to Lose Weight and Feel Great – Starting Today!

Copyright © 2016 by Katy Parsons

All rights Reserved. No part of this publication or the information in it may be quoted from or reproduced in any form by means such as printing, scanning, photocopying or otherwise without prior written permission of the copyright holder.

Disclaimer and Terms of Use

Please note the information contained within this document is for educational and entertainment purposes only. Every attempt has been made to provide accurate, up to date and reliable complete information. No warranties of any kind are expressed or implied. Readers acknowledge that the author is not engaging in the rendering of legal, financial, medical or professional advice. The content of this book has been derived from various sources. Please consult a licensed professional before attempting any techniques outlined in this book.

By reading this document, the reader agrees that under no circumstances is the author responsible for any losses, direct or indirect, which are incurred as a result of the use of information contained within this document, including, but not limited to, errors, omissions or inaccuracies.

The trademarks that are used are without any consent, and the publication of the trademark is without permissions or backing by the trademark owner. All trademarks and brands within this book are for clarifying purposes only and are the owned by the owners themselves, not affiliated with this document.

ISBN: 978-1-54-100144-2

First Edition: December 2016

10 9 8 7 6 5 4 3 2 1

Contents

Introduction viiii

Chapter 1: What is the Atkins Diet? 1
A Brief Overview of the Atkins Diet 2
Why Does it Work? 3
Ketosis Explained 4
Convinced That Atkins is for You? 5

Chapter 2: The Benefits of the Atkins Diet 7

Chapter 3: The Dos and Don'ts of the Atkins Diet 17
The Basics of the Atkins Diet 18
Do's and Don'ts 19
Common Atkins Diet Side Effects & How to Conquer Them! 20

Chapter 4: The Phases of the Atkins Diet 25
Phase 1 – Introduction Stage 25
Phase 2 – Food Induction 27
Phase 3 – Ongoing Weight Loss 28
Phase 4 – Maintenance 29
Don't Get Complacent! 31

Chapter 5: The Foods You Can And Can't Eat 33
Phase 1 34
Phase 2 37
Phase 3 38
Phase 4 38

Chapter 6: Phase 1 Meal Ideas, Two Weeks to Get You Started 41
Breakfast Ideas 42
Lunch ideas 42
Dinner ideas 43
A Few Snack Ideas 44
Sample Meal Plans 45

Points to Remember: *47*
The Advantages of Meal Planning *49*
The Importance of Exercise *50*

Chapter 7: The Emotional Side of Your Weight Loss Journey 53

Conclusion – Let's Sum It All Up! 59

Introduction

If you have ever attempted a diet, you will probably understand one word – hungry.

Most diets out there make you crave foods you can't have, you become hungry and irritated as a result, and you basically decide the whole thing isn't worth it and throw in the towel. What does this do? It creates a never ending circle of fad diets, lowering your self-esteem further and further, because you feel like you can't stick to it and you're not reaching your aims.

Put simply, the whole thing is a bit of a nightmare.

What if we told you that there was a diet out there that wouldn't leave you feeling hungry, where you could eat most of your favorite foods, and you would still lose a considerable amount of weight?

Seriously, we're not joking.

There's no red days and green days, no food weighing, and no major amount of counting involved either.

Again, we're really not joking.

Have you heard of the Atkins Diet?

You probably will have heard a lot about this diet, but you might not really understand what it really is. As with most things in life, the Atkins Diet has undergone a lot of changes over the last few years, developing from its original roots, and as a result, it is now easier to follow, more effective, and much more sustainable.

If you have picked up this book, that is probably because you are looking for a diet you can stick to without the usual pitfalls that other fad diets bring. The good news is that if you know how to use the Atkins Diet to its full potential, it can certainly work very well for you, without those painful hunger pangs, and the aforementioned throwing in the towel episodes.

We will talk in much more detail in our first full chapter about what the Atkins Diet is and how it works, and throughout this book we will give you all the important information you need on where to begin, what you can expect, the phases you will need to go through, what you can and can't eat, as well as meal plans to give you ideas and inspiration to begin. We will also give a nod to the emotional side of losing weight, because this is something you don't hear too much about.

Perhaps you think it's a ridiculous suggestion to say that there are any negative emotions connected to becoming healthier and slimmer, but you will certainly notice attitudes changing towards you, feelings within you changing, and all of this can be a little confusing; we will talk you through it all, so you know what to expect.

So, cast aside any ideas you might have about the Atkins Diet, clear your head and keep your mind open – we are about to take you on a journey to effective weight loss, a healthy lifestyle, and as a result, a much happier, and more slim-line you.

Chapter 1:
What is the Atkins Diet?

Around 10-15 years ago there were huge waves made by a new diet on the block, it was a diet which basically allowed you to eat all the foods that other diets said were unhealthy, and it also claimed to never let you feel hungry. Everyone wondered who on earth had come up with this crazy concept; surely this can't be true?

No, this is not a dream, this is a reality.

There was a lot of controversy about this diet, but that is probably because nobody could really get their heads around the scientific mechanics of it. The bottom line is that the Atkins Diet works, and it has been successful for millions of people across the globe. Yes, it has changed a lot since it was first developed back in 1972, by expert cardiologist Dr Robert C Atkins, but the changes have been even more positive, because today the diet is easier than ever to follow.

Okay, let's break it down into bite-sized chunks.

A Brief Overview of the Atkins Diet

The Atkins Diet was developed by, as we mentioned, a cardiologist called Robert C Atkins, hence the name. Dr Atkins realized that his patients could gain serious health benefits, as well as weight loss benefits, by cutting down the number of carbohydrates in their diet, and upping the amount of fat instead. That might sound like a ridiculous notion, but bear with us.

The Atkins Diet is a low carbohydrate diet, in fact let's not even call it a diet, because you're not actually restricting anything you will miss, let's call it an eating plan.

Yes, that sounds much better.

You are cutting down on the amount of carbohydrates in your diet, and instead you are eating more in the way of protein (very important for your body) and fats. Now, we know that lots of delicious foods have high fat content, and in this particular diet, sorry eating plan, you are therefore getting to eat the foods you enjoy – hence the lack of cravings. As we have mentioned before, probably one of the key reasons that people fall of the diet wagon is because of food cravings – when they are severe, you simply can't think of anything else, and the great thing about the Atkins Diet is that you simply won't have any.

The Atkins Diet (yes, we said eating plan, but you get the gist) has several stages, which we will discuss in much more detail in a later chapter dedicated to them. These stages are:

- Introduction
- Food induction
- Ongoing weight loss

- Maintenance

There are many companies out there who have done a twist on this theme and shows diets with more phases added, but the bottom line is that these are the basics of the diet, and if you choose to add in the extra phase here and there, you're probably just complicating matters. Why give yourself a bigger headache than you need to?

The first phase starts with more restriction of carbs, and as you move through the phases, you slowly reintroduce a higher level of carbs, until your body reaches a point where it maintains your weight loss, without piling the pounds back on. If you find you do start to see a creeping gain, you simply start back at phase one. Easy.

Why Does it Work?

You're probably a little confused at this stage about how something that sounds too good to be true actually works, but it's all about making your body think in a different way. You're actually tricking your body in some ways, being sneaky, but it certainly works.

Let's get a little scientific.

The rate at which you burn food is called your metabolism, and everyone's metabolism works at different rates. The key to understanding weight loss is really about understanding your metabolism, but that is a very complicated subject to get into. Basically, in the regular run of things, you burn carbs for energy, and you get carbs from carbohydrate-rich food and sugar. Carbs are turned into sugar by the body, and then this sugar is used as fuel to give you the energy to go about your daily business and for your body to run effectively. Now, if you burn sugar for energy, you're not affecting your existing fat stores, they just sit there, all wobbly and annoying.

On the other hand, if you limit the amount of carbs you consume, your body is forced into something called ketosis. Don't worry, ketosis is not dangerous provided it is done in the correct way, and the Atkins Diet makes sure this happens.

A regular diet restricts calories but remains high in carbs, and that is why you get sugar highs and lows, which result in bad moods, tiredness, and, you guessed it, hunger pangs and cravings.

If you've ever been on a diet before you will know that hunger pangs are *the worst*.

As a result, this type of diet is just not sustainable.

Are you with us so far?

Okay, now the Atkins Diet works by using fat for energy, rather than carbs. You are using the fat from the foods you eat, as well as the fat you have been storing (remember, that wobbly, annoying fat we just mentioned? You're going to get rid of that much more easily) – all of this results in weight loss. You are also eating more calories in effect, so you don't get those hunger pangs, episodes of tiredness, or bad, irritable moods.

You basically lose weight but feel full, all because of this thing called ketosis.

Ketosis Explained

Probably the most confusing part of the Atkins Diet is understanding what ketosis actually is. It's really not that difficult once you realize what it is, what it does, and you are reassured that it isn't dangerous.

Ketosis is a natural bodily function, it is a metabolic state, and it is usually referred to in diabetes management. That's not to say that ketosis doesn't have a role to play in other areas of the body, and weight loss is certainly one of them.

You will probably have heard of the Keto Diet, or the Paleo Diet, and these two both use ketosis as the main staying point of the diets, but the difference with the Atkins Diet is that it really only fully utilises ketosis for the first phase; after that you are slowly reintroducing carbs, gently taking your body out of ketosis, or only just keeping it on the cusp.

When your body isn't receiving enough carbs to burn for energy it switches its thinking and goes to burn fat instead. As we talked about earlier, if you burn fat for energy, you are eating into your fat stores, and this is a much more effective way to lose weight, give yourself less of a hungry feeling, and feel more energised, because you are still getting energy from the calories you aren't restricting in your diet.

When the body switches to burning fat, it begins to produce something called ketones, and this is a normal process, not harmful, and provided you keep your intake of protein within the recommended amount, your body will function normally, effectively, and actually, in a much healthier way.

So, to give it a much more basic explanation – ketosis is simply changing how your body thinks.

Convinced That Atkins is for You?

Hopefully by this point you will be ready and raring to go, eager to start your journey towards weight loss. The point of this diet is that you really won't feel like you're actually on a diet, because it lacks the distinct feel of one – i.e. you won't be hungry!

Think of the Atkins Diet as a bit of a food-fest, you can eat and feel full, lose weight, have more energy, and basically fit into those clothes that you've been eyeing up in your wardrobe for the last year or so.

If you're convinced (and if not, why not), then read on to find out more about this highly effective, and easy to follow diet.

Chapter 2:
The Benefits of the Atkins Diet

We have talked in our first chapter about what the Atkins Diet is, and how it is easy to follow, with great results. Now, we really need to give you an overview of its benefits, because nobody on this planet does anything without it having a major benefit to it!

Over the years there have been many studies into how low carb diets overall work, and how they can benefit, or perhaps even hinder, the body. The results of these studies have certainly come out in the favor of these types of diets, and the Atkins Diet has been shown to be one of the most effective, not only in terms of losing weight and looking super slim, but for many other health issues too.

You can break these down really into two separate sections – the weight loss and appearance side of it, and the more deeply hidden health benefits.

Let's check them out one by one.

Less cravings than other diets

We have touched upon this already in our first section, but it is probably the number one reason why people stick with this diet, because you don't have that hideous hunger feeling that many other diets give you. Low carb diets, such as the Atkins Diet, but also the Keto Diet, and the Paleo Diet too, are obviously low in carbohydrate intake, and that means your blood sugar levels are kept much more even as a result of not eating as many carbs. A low calorie and high carb diet gives you those sugar highs and lows, which result in bad moods, poor focus and concentration, and those aforementioned cravings that have you raiding the fridge and biscuit tin in desperation.

Come on, you've done it before, everyone has!

This simply makes you feel terrible that you have fallen off your diet wagon, but if you stick to the low carb ethos of the Atkins Diet, you have steadier blood sugar levels, and that means no highs and lows, and less cravings as a result. You are less hungry because you are eating protein-rich foods and fats, which are known to keep you fuller for longer, and be generally more satisfying, so you are full, but you lose weight.

Number one reason most people go with the Atkin's Diet, it has to be said!

Guaranteed weight loss

Because you are making your body think in a totally different way (e.g. you are sending it into ketosis), you are going to lose weight, 100% guaranteed. Those fat stores which are usually untouched on a regular low calorie diet are burnt away, and that means you will probably have bigger losses, much quicker. Your mood is going to soar high as a result, your confidence will be instantly on the up, and generally speaking, you're going to feel lighter and healthier.

The downside? You're probably going to need to buy new clothes, or a whole new wardrobe, but that's hardly a terrible side effect, right?

Reduction in acne symptoms

There has been some evidence to show that followers of the Atkins Diet reported a reduction in acne symptoms, helping to clear up the skin and prevent flare ups and break outs. Why? It is probably because you are making healthier food choices, e.g. less carbs and sugars, but whatever the science behind it, it's a major benefit for anyone who has been upset by this condition in the past.

You can find out your 'happy weight', so you maintain your loss

When you have reached a weight that you are happy with, you can easily maintain it by using the Atkins Diet phases to test it out. You are teaching your body to basically survive on a different level of carbohydrate intake than it has been used to, and you need to find the level at which your body can run on, without either losing weight, or gaining it either. If you find you are creeping back up on the scales, then you simply return to phase one and try again, until you find that happy weight you and your internal body are satisfied with.

Many diets out there work for the short-term, but as soon as you start eating properly again, everything piles back on and you wonder why you bothered wasting your time and effort; the Atkins Diet is different because it allows you to maintain much easier – this is no crash diet!

You are encouraged to make healthier food choices, which become habit after a short time

By taking more notice of what you eat and the way your body handles it, you will instantly start to make much healthier choices. For instance, you will focus much more on vitamins and minerals, rather than the stuff out there that is bad for you, so you're a healthier individual as a result.

You lose fat from the places you want to

Okay ladies, let's be honest here (sorry guys, but this starting point really is for the ladies) – how many times have you been on a diet and you see the scales going down (and you're hungry, very, very hungry), but the only difference in the mirror is from the places you *really* didn't want to lose it from, such as your breasts and face. Sounds familiar?

Of course, guys you can resonate with this too, because you may find you have a bit of a beer belly appearing, but you try and diet and it doesn't disappear from there at first. Annoying, isn't it?

This is because we have two different types of fat in our body, and the regular low-calorie diets out there tend to focus on the wrong type. Where you store fat in your body really tells you how healthy or otherwise you are, and how much of a risk you have in terms of serious disease, such as heart issues, diabetes, and stroke. We have subcutaneous fat, and we have visceral fat; subcutaneous fat is stored under the skin, but visceral fat is the type you want to try and reduce, but this builds up around organs, and drive up blood pressure, increase cholesterol, block arteries, and basically causes chaos.

The Atkins Diet, being low in carbs, uses up fat stores for energy, as we have mentioned, and that means your visceral fat stores are being targeted, essentially cutting your chances of developing serious illness in the future. On a vainer note, you're basically going to look slimmer in the places you want to look slimmer!

Studies have shown epilepsy sufferers can gain benefit from low carb diets

Whilst there is some question mark over why and how, studies have shown that low carb diets, such as the Atkins Diet, can help epilepsy suffers with their symptoms, and therefore reduce the severity of the condition, when used in conjunction with regular medication.

Less chance of developing diabetes in the future

Prevention of diabetes is a very real benefit of the Atkins Diet, and it has a lot to do with that process we were talking about earlier – ketosis. When you lower the amount of carbs you eat in your diet, you are also lowering the amount of insulin that your body needs to produce. This all works hand in hand with your chances of developing type I or II diabetes at some point in the future, because your insulin levels are not spiking, and instead, they are kept very steady indeed.

Hello good cholesterol, goodbye bad cholesterol!

We have two types of cholesterol in our body, and we need both to function healthily; having said that, we obviously need less of the bad, and more of the good. The good type is called HDL, and this carries cholesterol away from the body, and into the liver, where it is processed and then either recycled, or it is gotten rid of completely. Now, on the other hand, LDL is the bad guy, because this type carries cholesterol *from* the liver, into and around the rest of the body.

The only way to up your levels of the good stuff and lower your levels of the bad stuff is to eat more fat, and we know that with the Atkins Diet, the focus is on exactly that.

Lower blood pressure, less chance of heart disease and stroke

Eating less carbs has been shown to lower your blood pressure, and we all know that raised blood pressure, or hypertension to give it its medical name, can drastically increase your chances of developing heart disease, having a heart attack, or having a stroke.

Basically, we could put many symptoms under an umbrella here, including less chance of diabetes, lower blood pressure, reduced obesity, and lower cholesterol levels – these are all immediately helped by the Atkins Diet, simply because you are in ketosis, and not eating as many carbs.

Better sleep quality

Going to bed hungry is no fun, in fact going to bed hungry is not a great recipe for a good night's sleep! If you've ever had a rather terrible night of tossing and turning, you will understand that a) you're really not good for anything the next day, b) you're not going to be in the best of moods, causing everyone to avoid you like the plague, and c) you're probably going to want to eat everything in sight as a result. Having a much more even blood sugar level, whilst feeling full and satisfied, is basically going to help you nod off to sleep much easier, and could also help you sustain your sleep until the morning, leaving you feeling well-rested and happier overall.

You will feel full of energy, ready to run that marathon ... or perhaps something less strenuous!

Okay, so maybe you're not going to feel like you're ready to do the next long distance marathon, but you will feel full of energy to get you through your working day, without those energy slumps that you might have suffered with before. Feeling hungry does not help you concentrate, and if you can't concentrate, you're simply going to get fidgety, tired, and you're going to make unhealthy food choices in terms of snacking on the wrong things. The Atkins Diet helps you feel more evenly fuelled, without highs and lows, so as a result your energy levels will stay steady, without slumps.

Better concentration and focus

If you have more energy and you're not thinking too much about the things you want to eat and can't, you're going to be able to focus much better than you would do otherwise. On top of this, the Atkins Diet has been shown to boost your overall focus and concentration levels, because eating a diet which is more satisfying, e.g. protein and fat, helps fuel your body consistently, and we know that you don't only need to fuel your body but your mind too.

There has actually been some suggestion that low carb diets overall can help cut your chances of developing conditions such as Alzheimer's and Parkinson's, and slow down the condition if you already have it. Whilst there is ongoing research going into this, the signs which have come out of these studies so far have been extremely heartening and encouraging. This is because there is a very strong connection between the foods you eat and the development of conditions such as Alzheimer's, whilst also being very strongly connected with diabetes – obviously we know that the Atkins Diet is very effective at cutting your chances of developing diabetes, whilst also helping to steady blood sugar and help regulate insulin production.

Better mood – nobody wants to be around a grouch

If you're tired, hungry, and lacking in energy, are you going to be a fun, happy person? Probably not. If you've ever been on a restrictive diet before, you will probably have found that you were not full of the joys of life at that particular time, because you were too busy dreaming about chocolate. So, if you're not hungry, and you're not feeling tired, all because you're full and satisfied, without feeling too restricted, you're going to be much more pleasant and fun to be around, right?

Do your friends and family a favor, cut out the grouchiness!

As you can see, the Atkins Diet has plentiful benefits, both for your body, mind, and your general appearance. Of course, your mood is also advantageous for those around you too!

Whilst we can't avoid the fact that the Atkins Diet has courted negative press in the past, we should also point out that much of this is because nobody really understood the mechanics of it at the time. Can something so good really be true?

Well, in this case yes it can, and you can see that from the sheer number of benefits we've listed and talked about one by one.

So, we know what the Atkins Diet is, and we know how it can benefit us, but in our next chapter we're going to go into a little more detail on how it actually works. Yes, we talked about it to some degree in our first chapter, but if you're going to embark on a journey of this scale, you really need to make sure you understand it totally – reiteration never hurt anyone!

Let's move on with our journey.

Chapter 3:
The Dos and Don'ts of the Atkins Diet

We are talking about your body, and essentially that means we are talking about your life – for that reason, it's important that you understand completely what you're letting yourself in for, and that means you understand more than completely how this whole thing works.

You should never jump feet first into anything you don't really 'get', and the aim of this book overall is to help you understand the path you're going down, and the mechanics behind it. If you are at this point in our book and you still don't really understand how the Atkins Diet works, or you're just not convinced that something so easy can be true, then the best advice is to head back to chapter one and go over it again; by this point you should understand how it works at least.

Now, even if you get the mechanics of it, you need to know the common pitfalls that could come your way, before we really go into exactly how to follow the diet. Consider this chapter your troubleshooting 101, giving you all the hints and tips you need to jump over any potential hurdles, with all that extra energy you'll have!

The Basics of the Atkins Diet

We talked about the diet and how it works in short terms in our first chapter, but let's go over the basics again, before we get into a bit more detail. In very short and easy to understand points:

- The Atkins Diet is a low carbohydrate diet
- Other diets which are similar in some ways to the Atkins Diet include the Keto Diet (Ketogenic), and the Paleo Diet
- The Atkins Diet uses a metabolic state which is naturally occurring within the body to change the way it thinks, and the way it fuels, called ketosis
- Whilst regular low calorie diets burn carbs for fuel, the Atkins Diet burns fats for fuel, which means it is eating into your existing fat stores, helping you lose weight faster
- The Atkins Diet also helps keep your blood sugar levels regular and steady, without cravings and hunger
- You will move through set phases to complete the diet correctly
- There are many health benefits to the Atkins Diet, which have been proven in studies

Okay, that's the basics, and in the coming chapters we're going to tell you exactly what you can and can't eat (this is a diet, you can't just eat everything!), as well as give you some meal plans to show you some inspiration on your daily chow downs, but for now, this is exactly what you should and shouldn't do when following the Atkins Diet.

Do's and Don'ts

- **Do count net carbs** – During the first phase of the Atkins Diet in particular, you need to count your carb intake quite strictly. This is because in the first stage, you need to make sure your body is well and truly in ketosis, and not teetering on the edge – teetering is not good! One of the biggest mistakes people make is to measure total carbs, and this is incorrect – you need to measure net carbs per day. You can easily find an online carb calculator to help you with this, and keep a track as the day goes on.
- **Do drink plenty of water** – Too many people make the big common error of not drinking enough water, but the bottom line is that you need to glug the H2O because your body needs it! During the first stages of ketosis your body uses up stored fluid and that can leave you dehydrated if you don't replenish what you're losing. On top of this, you will notice the rather inconvenient side effect during the first week or so of needing to go to the toilet to pee quite a lot! Of course, you're losing fluids by doing this, so make sure you drink water to stay hydrated.
- **Do keep your salt intake up** – When you lose water, you lose minerals, and you need to keep salting your food to make sure you replenish it. Of course, don't go overboard, but generally speaking, on any low carb diet, salt is not a bad thing. If you are on any medication for high blood pressure, or even low blood pressure, check this out with your doctor first.
- **Do make sure you eat the recommended amount of protein** – Depending on whether you are male or

female, and your height, you need to make sure you eat the recommended amount of protein for you. This is because protein and fat are the main stays of the Atkins Diet, and if you don't eat protein, or not enough, you're not going to feel full, and then you're going to get cravings; if that's the case, it's just not going to work.

- **Don't weigh yourself every day** – It's important to realize that your natural weight is going to fluctuate on a daily basis, and if you weigh yourself every single day, for reassurance or some other reason, you're just setting yourself up for failure and upset. Give yourself one day a week when you weigh yourself, perhaps a Sunday, and do it first thing in the morning when you've been to the toilet, and take all your clothes off too. That is your guideline.
- **Don't forget to track your diet** – Creating a diet diary is a great tool for motivation, but it is also good way to find areas where you could improve and do better. Treat yourself to a fancy new notebook and make it your journal to success!
- **Don't forget to check food labels** – Just because an item says it's half fat or low calorie, it doesn't mean that it is lacking in carbs. There are many sneaky carbs out there, so get au fait with food labels and know what to look for, tying this in with your daily amount.

Common Atkins Diet Side Effects & How to Conquer Them!

We need to address the fact that there may be a transitional period which your body needs to go through before the plain sailing can begin. This is normal, any adjustment will throw up a few issues, and whilst the potential side effects of the Atkins

Diet at first aren't particular terrible, they can be a little annoying to deal with, until they pass.

The good news is that any side effects you develop will pass, and it is simply because your body is adjusting to ketosis. Remember, ketosis is not the usual run of the mill functioning method for your body, it is a metabolic state it goes into under duress or other circumstances, so you need to give your body a little slack until it gets used to it. Think about when you start a new job for instance, at first you're not firing on all cylinders, but after a few weeks you have it nailed, and you can begin to coast your way through your working day – your body is the same when it first starts the Atkins Diet.

Of course, if you find any symptoms are prolonged, it doesn't hurt to go and have a chat with your doctor, just to check things out, but overall, any side effects should pass after a short time.

In this section we will run through the common side effects of the Atkins Diet, in fact the common side effects of any low carb diet, and we will also give you the information you need on how to overcome them – good news! They can be overcome! The key thing to remember here however is patience – think of the bigger picture.

Okay, so what the common side effects?

- **Going to the toilet to pee – a lot** - This is normal, and as we mentioned in our section about eating salt and drinking plenty of water, it is your body using up your fluid stores in the first part of ketosis. As you use up these stores you are also kicking them out, and that is why you need to pee a little more than normal. It's important to remember that this could leave you dehydrated if you don't put back what you're losing, so make sure you drink plenty of water, and make sure you eat enough salt, to avoid mineral loss. Your kidneys are going to be producing more water at this stage too, which is another reason for this rather annoying side effect. Probably the best advice is also to never be too far away from the toilet! Again, this will pass after a short time.

- **Dizziness and lethargy** – Whilst your body is figuring out what is going on, there is going to be a period of time where you may feel a little dizzy and you may feel more tired than normal. Again, this is quite common and it will pass over time. It is thought that this particular side effect is down to mineral loss again, so perhaps the best way to conquer it is to go down the line of salt once more! Pack your diet with leafy vegetables wherever possible, and dairy too, as these are high in the mineral you need – potassium. This will give you more in the way of energy and it will also help with any dizziness issues.
- **Headaches** – This is probably the most common side effect you will experience, and provided the headaches aren't prolonged or extremely severe, you can rest safe in the knowledge that this phase will pass. The development of headaches is again all down to mineral loss, and if you can remember to salt everything and try and pack in potassium-rich foods, whilst also drinking plenty of water, you notice that the headaches drastically improve as you get into the diet.
- **Cravings, but only at first** – For a very short time at the start of the diet, you *may* notice some slight cravings. As

soon as you start eating properly into the diet you will notice these disappear completely, and again, this is a very short lived potential side effect, in fact, not everyone even notices this problem. The reason for it is that your body is figuring out what is going on, and that can send everything a little bit loca for a short time; don't worry, it will pass very quickly.

- **Muscle cramps** – Yet again, this is down to mineral loss! You'll probably have noticed by now that this is the main problem with the start of the Atkins Diet, but this is also a common theme in any low carb diet, and can easily be sorted out. Yet again, salt is your ally, and water is also. It's true that cramping muscles can be painful, but this certainly shouldn't last for too long and provided you go down the salt and water route, you should be able to minimize it quite easily.
- **Sleep pattern upset** – Again, this is down to your body being a little up in the air for a short time, and that can also affect your sleep patterns slightly. Basically you need to relax as much as possible before you sleep, maybe enjoy a warm drink, and you should be able to nod off a little easier. The good news is that once the effects of the diet kick in, you'll be sleeping like a baby every night anyway!

Side effects are quite a personal deal, so if you're not getting anything like the above list, and you're sailing through the first stage of heading into ketosis, well, well done you! If you're suffering from a few or all of them, be reassured that it's normal, and it will settle down quite quickly once your body figures out what the hell is going on.

Probably the most important thing to state at this point is that you really shouldn't be put off trying the Atkins Diet because we've told you about a few potential side effects. The key word there is 'potential', they are certainly not definite, and even if you get them, or just a few of them, they are not debilitating in any way, shape, or form, and will pass quickly. There is no diet out there which is without side effects, and if anyone tells you about one, they are lying! Your body is learning to think in a different way, and this is a process, something you need to adjust to. Once the transition is over, you really are into smooth sailing, all the way to a much healthier, and slim-line version of who you are now.

It's very important to understand exactly how to follow the Atkins Diet, because deviating from it is going to affect the way your body works. Ketosis is a metabolic state, we've mentioned this several times, and once you send your body into this state, it's important to avoid confusing matters; if your body has just gone through the transition process, you don't want to be throwing it a curveball, because all that is going to happen is you're going to get more side effects, you're going to not lose weight, and the chances are you might even put weight on.

Be sure about what you need to do before you begin, reading every point in this book until you understand it. Our coming chapters will give you much more in-depth information about exactly what to do on this diet, including what you can and (unfortunately) can't eat.

So, without further ado, let's check out the phases of the Atkins Diet.

Chapter 4:
The Phases of the Atkins Diet

The Atkins Diet is, in its most basic form, a 4 phase diet, but you will notice if you Google it that there are companies out there who will claim to have diets with up to 14 phases – do you really need to add complication to your diet? No!

Stick to these 4 phases and you will certainly see the differences you are aiming for, without complicating your mind and getting confused. If you confuse matters too much, you risk following the diet incorrectly, and as we mentioned at the end of our last chapter, if you follow the diet and make mistakes, you're not going to get the benefits you're wanting.

If you're going to do something, at least do it right!

Okay, so let's check out the 4 phases of the Atkins Diet.

Phase 1 – Introduction Stage

The first stage of the Atkins Diet is when you are more likely to notice side effects of some sort, and as we talked about at length in our last chapter, this is because your body is trying to figure out what is happening. You have suddenly started eating in a different way, and as a result it needs to switch its fuel sources to make sure it is getting what it needs. Give your body a little slack here, it might be extremely clever, but it is not a genius! A short time is all it will need to figure it out and start running in tip top condition again. Don't be thinking that this particular stage is unhealthy however, because as we have said time and time again, ketosis is a naturally occurring metabolic state, and provided you follow the rules of this phase, there is nothing dangerous about it.

Okay, warning over. This particular phase is the most restrictive in terms of how many carbs you can eat. You need to be restrictive here because you need to force your body into that initial ketosis, and if you eat too many it's just going to grab onto the carbs you do eat, and use them as fuel instead. Obviously, this is not what we want – we want to be using fats for fuel instead.

Download a good quality carb calculator to help with your counting here, so you don't go wrong without realizing it. It's also important to understand food labels at this stage too, because there are many hidden carbs you need to avoid.

Key points in phase 1:

- You are allowed a daily amount of 20g of carbs
- You should not go below 18g of carbs
- Do not go over 22g under any circumstances
- Phase 1 should last for around 2 weeks on average
- You should stage in phase 1 until you are 15lb from your ideal goal body weight

- You can stay in this phase for longer than 2 weeks if you want to lose a lot of weight fast, however exercise caution
- Make sure you have 4-6oz of protein each day
- Don't forget that you need to eat fat, because this is what you are going to be burning for energy
- Aim to eat three meals per day, with two snacks in-between
- Don't forget to drink plenty of water and salt your meals

You can easily load your diet at this stage with as much meat, fish, fats, eggs, vegetables, and poultry as you like, in fact you are encouraged to eat until you are full! How many diets do you know that say that? Check out some Atkins Diet cookbooks for inspiration on what to eat.

Phase 2 – Food Induction

The second stage of the diet involves you slowly increasing your carb intake on a daily basis, and again, it's a good idea to use a carb calculator here, to make sure you don't undo your good work in phase 1, by accidentally eating too many carbs. Again, you can eat until you are full.

By the time you reach phase 2, the idea is that you will have probably lost more than half of the weight you wanted, and this is the beginning of slowly introducing your body back into the idea of eating carbs, but still burning fats for fuel. You need to go slowly at this stage, because you are nursing your body back from the ketosis of stage 1, so give your internal system a little slack here still.

Key points in phase 2:

- If you want to lose your weight in a more steady manner, you can simply follow phase 1 for the recommended 2 weeks, and then head into phase 2 for a slower rate of weight loss
- Add into your diet foods such as nuts, seeds, fruits, cottage cheese, yogurt etc
- Phase 2 is about maintaining and moving forwards, not going backward, so keep an eye on the scales, however only do this once per week to avoid noticing normal bodily fluctuations
- You should generally stage in phase 2 until you are around 10lb away from your goal
- You are allowed 25g of carbs per day

By the time you are firmly in phase 2, you will notice that the initial side effects you noticed in the first stage should have gone, or at least drastically improved.

Phase 3 – Ongoing Weight Loss

The aim is that by the end of phase 3, you will have reached your goal, and you can then go onto the final phase of the diet, which is all about maintaining your good work and finding out your body's own personal carb level. This particular phase is about finishing off what you have started and again, the theme is about increasing your carb intake a little further. Weight loss will slow down as you move through the phases, from a more dramatic loss in phase 1, a slightly lower rate in phase 2, and even slower again in phase 3, but that's perfectly fine, because the scales are definitely moving downwards, you're considerably slimmer than when you started, and you're bouncing around with extra energy, happiness, and ultra-body confidence!

Key points in phase 3:

- You should remain on phase 3 until you have reached your goal and stayed there for around one month without budging. This means you have found your body's own personal carb intake level of tolerance
- You are allowed 35g of carbs per day, but if you find that you are starting to gain a little, try working at 30g for a short time, and then increasing up to 35g slowly
- This phase should help you understand the way your body works, because you are fine tuning your personal tolerance to carbs, understanding which foods work for you, and which don't
- If you find you hit a brick wall in terms of weight loss, drop your carb intake back to 30g, before moving back to 35g a week or two later

You are now virtually at the end of the Atkins Diet by this stage, because phase 4 is more about lifetime maintenance than tweaking a diet. You are now aware of what your body likes and doesn't like in terms of weight gain or loss, and it's important to realize that this is entirely personal – just because your friend can eat a certain food and not budge on the scales at all, doesn't mean you can! We are all individual and our diets and lifestyles should reflect this; there is no use in moaning and getting upset because you can't eat your body weight in chocolate without breaking out in spots and piling on the pounds, just because your friend down the road can do that once a month and only put 1lb on – he/she is lucky, and karma will catch up!

Phase 4 – Maintenance

First things first, by this stage you should be patting yourself on the back big time and saying 'well done me!' You have lost the weight you wanted to lose, you are new and slinky, and you are also healthier as a result. You will be noticing all the visible differences, but you will also be noticing a lot of internal differences too, especially about confidence and the way you view yourself.

Seriously, at this stage, allow yourself to be self-indulgent and big yourself up!

The hard work isn't finished however, because now you need to maintain what you have achieved, and this is really down to continuing the rest of your life in a healthy manner, and not falling back into the unhealthy practices that you may have done before.

By this phase you know what you can and can't eat without noticing a massive difference in the scales, and you should also understand that you should only weigh yourself once per week, simply to keep an eye on things.

Key points in phase 4

- This particular phase goes on for the rest of your life
- You are now the captain of your carb steering ship, because you now know how much in the way of carbs your body can handle, and you should stick to that
- If you find you are putting weight on, you can reduce your carb level down slightly, by 5g, and then check the difference, if you are still gaining, reduce it by another 5g – never go below the phase 1 amount however, and avoid going that low unless you need to at this point

- Turn this phase into your healthy lifestyle – remember to exercise regularly, drink plenty of water, watch your diet intake, and only drink alcohol in moderation

Having worked through the Atkins Diet and its four main stages, you now have all the information and armory you need to continue your life at the goal weight you have achieved. You have also learned a lot about your body and nutrition, which is something you should never allow yourself to forget.

Don't Get Complacent!

Just a word of warning.

Of course, you should be extremely proud of yourself, but you should also not allow yourself to get complacent and simply slip back into your old habits. If you do this, you will notice a drastic weight gain and you have undone all the work you tirelessly put in whilst you were following the phases of the Atkins Diet.

Always remember how hard you worked, and if it helps, keep a before and after photo of yourself somewhere handy, just to give yourself a prompt reminder.

In our next two chapters we will give you plenty of ideas on the foods you can and can't eat, as well as meals plans to throw some inspiration into the air.

Chapter 5: The Foods You Can And Can't Eat

Every diet has a set of foods which you can eat to your heart's content, a set which you should be careful of, and a set which you should avoid under all circumstances, this is simply the law of diets. If you are looking for a particular diet which lets you eat whatever the hell you like, as often as you like, well, you're going to be looking for a long time!

The great thing about the Atkins Diet is that it doesn't restrict the foods that all too often you seriously crave when you're on a calorie restrictive diet, which is what leads to less in the way of cravings and sugar crashes. Throughout this chapter we are going to be talking about the foods you can and can't eat during each phase of the Atkins Diet. Remember from reading out last chapter that the particular phases of this diet are there to be personalised for you, and you can choose to stay in each phase for as long as you need – everyone's metabolism is different, everyone's weight loss aim is different, and therefore everyone's Atkins Diet path is slightly different too.

Remember to keep your intake of protein within the recommended amount, which currently stands at 0.8g of protein per kg of your body. For the average man this generally means around 56g per day, but you should certainly check your particular weight in terms of how much you should be eating. Protein is vital in the Atkins Diet, because it gives you the energy and muscle strength you need to function. You should also not be scared of eating fats! Remember that we are wanting to burn fat for energy, so you need to keep your intake high in order to have enough energy to get through the day, and to allow the important functions of your organs to take place.

You should also check out online recipes dedicated to the Atkins Diet, because this will help give you plentiful variety in your diet, without boredom creeping in.

Okay, let's check out each phase and what you can and can't eat.

Phase 1

Remember, eat until you are full! At this stage you are restricting your carb intake to 20g.

You can eat …

- Any type of fish, such as tuna, cod, halibut, herring, sardines, trout etc
- Any type of poultry, such as chicken, duck, pheasant, turkey, ostrich, quail etc
- Any shellfish, such as shrimp, squid, lobster, crab – one point to remember here is that oysters and mussels have a significant carb level compared to the rest, so be

careful how much you eat here, using your carb calculator to keep track.

- Any meat, including bacon, beef, lamb, ham, pork, veal, venison etc. Meat makes up a huge part of the Atkins Diet so you need to chow on down, however do be careful of processed types of meat, such as bacon, because it can be cured with sugars which can give you extra towards your carb intake amount for that particular day. Again, use your carb calculator and check food labels.
- Eggs, however you like them!
- Any type of fat, and any type of oil – this can include butter, mayonnaise, and any type of vegetable oil
- Cheese, any type you like. Remember that some cheeses do have a carb amount so you will need to add this to your allowance for the day, but it is very minimal, and you can safely have around 3-4oz per day in whatever way you like.
- Vegetables – throw them into your diet and make sure you get your daily amount of vitamins and minerals. It's a good guideline to simply have a portion of vegetable with every meal in some guise, however again, be aware that some vegetables contain carbs, albeit a small amount, such as mushrooms, broccoli and olives etc. Tomatoes in particular are quite high in terms of carb content when compared to other fruits and vegetables, but provided you add this to your allowance, you're fine.
- Herbs and spices – Use to season your food to your heart's content.
- Beverages – Make sure you drink plenty of water, as we have discussed previously, and this can be filtered, mineral, tap, or spring water. If you are a coffee fan, you

can still drink caffeinated coffee, but limit it to one or two cups per day; the same goes for tea. If you go for diet soda drinks, beware that they do contain carbs, so add this to your daily amount.

We can't give you an exhaustive list of what you can and can't eat here, because we would be going all day long, but the fact remains that in this stage you simply need to make sure you are getting your protein amount and that you count your carb intake so that it doesn't go over 20g – this is the most restrictive stage in terms of carbs, as we have mentioned time and time again.

With that in mind, what you basically need to avoid is anything which is high in carbs, so in this phase, avoid like the plague the following:

- Fruit
- Bread
- Anything containing grains
- Vegetables which are starchy
- Alcohol
- Dairy products, apart from cheese and butter

Probably the hardest part of this phase is the fact that you can't eat bread. Most of us will admit to loving bread in some guise, and giving it up completely is imperative in this phase. Bread is a living, breathing carb, and this phase is about avoiding high carb foods. Sorry, but your bread addiction is going to need to be conquered if you're going to do well in phase 1!

Okay, now we know what we can and can't eat in phase 1, and we're well on the road to checking out creative recipes to pull it all together, let's look at phase 2.

Phase 2

The next phase means you can slowly reintroduce some carbs into your diet, going up by 5g per day. Now, this certainly doesn't give you free rein, but it does give you a little more freedom. Remember to check your carb allowance against the net carbs that you are allowed, to keep yourself within limits.

In phase 2, you can eat the following;

- Dairy products, including mozzarella cheese, ricotta cheese, cottage cheese, yogurt, whole milk, and cream
- Nuts and seeds, any you like. Be careful of peanuts, pecans and cashews however, as these have a higher carb content than the others
- Fruits – This is perhaps the biggest reintroduction you can make, because at this stage you are allowed a certain amount of fruit, such as blackberries, strawberries, honey-dew melon, and cranberries. Avoid the exotic fruits during phase 2, as they are higher in sugars, and therefore higher in carbs
- Lemon, lime, and tomato juice
- Beans and lentils
- On the go microwave meals – check the carb content on the back of the box and subtract it from your carb allowance for that day.

Remember:

Obviously, you can still eat anything from phase 1 in addition to these foods listed here; what you see here is simply what can be slowly reintroduced into your diet, always keep chowing down on meat, fish, eggs etc, as you did in phase 1.

Phase 3

This particular phase, as we talked about in our phases chapter, is about adding a little more in the way of carbs to your diet from what you had before. At this stage, you are allowed 35g of carbs per day. Remember, you can eat anything from our phase 1 list, and you should make sure you get your full quota of protein per day, plus making sure you get enough fat in your diet too. In this phase you can add in the following foods, within your carb allowance.

- Vegetables which are starchy, but more variety, including carrots, beets, peas, sweet potato, regular potato, and corn
- More fruits, including exotic fruits, such as coconut, cherries, watermelon, papaya, guava, apple, kiwi, grapefruit, apricot, pineapple, mango, peach, grapes, orange, banana, date, and pears
- Grains, including wheat germ, oat bran, quinoa, whole wheat bread, oatmeal, polenta, whole wheat pasta, oatmeal, barley, brown rice

Bread at last! By phase 3 you can start to reintroduce bread in small amounts, but avoid the white sort, you should always go for whole wheat for a simple healthy reason.

Phase 4

By this phase you can basically eat normally, provided you keep an eye on your cab intake, and you stick to the level that your body works well at. Throughout the Atkins Diet you will have realized the tolerance level to which your body works in conjunction with carbs, and when you go over that level, you will begin to put on weight; obviously vice versa, if you go under it, you will lose weight. Stick to your happy level and you will maintain.

The key thing to remember – phase 4 is your eating plan for the rest of your life, so keep it varied, keep it on target, and remember to load up your diet with healthy fruits and vegetables, as well as your daily allowance of protein, and your happy level of carbs.

We won't go on to list everything you can eat in phase 4, because it should be pretty obvious!

So, there it is, your list of what you can and can't eat during the Atkins Diet. It's not as bad as you thought, is it! See, sometimes the thinking can be worse than reality, and you can now see that the Atkins Diet is really not that restrictive at all. Probably the hardest part of it is phase 1, and probably the cutting out of bread. If you can learn to live without bread, you will feel much less bloated, and you will instantly notice a difference in the way you feel overall.

To pull all of this together, our next chapter is going to give you some meal ideas, to help you put some variation into your diet, as well as helping you get started during the first two weeks of your phase 1 plan.

Chapter 6:
Phase 1 Meal Ideas, Two Weeks to Get You Started

It's all very well and good saying 'this is phase 1, this is what you can eat, and this is what you shouldn't eat', but how do you pull it all together to give you an actionable plan for the first phase of your diet? The Atkins Diet isn't rocket science, but when you're trying to get your head around something new, all the help you can get is preferable!

In this chapter we're going to give you a big helping hand, and we're going to give you a two weeks' of meal ideas to get you through the first section of your diet. We did mention previously that you can continue on phase 1 for longer than two weeks if you want to, but generally speaking, this set fortnight will be enough for a regular amount of weight loss. If you want to stay in this phase for longer, by the end of two weeks you will have lots more ideas on what to eat, and how to mix it all up.

So, let's give you a few ideas of meals you can eat during the first phase of your Atkins journey.

Breakfast Ideas

- Cheese omelet with onions and mushrooms
- Mexican breakfast peppers – Simply stuff a large pepper with pork and beef chorizo, onions, cheddar cheese and egg
- Turkey sausage with red and green peppers (sauté)
- Buttermilk cinnamon waffles
- Baked eggs with cheese – Just bake eggs, cream, and cheese in the oven)
- Corned beef hash
- Scrambled eggs with spinach
- Stuffed Portobello mushrooms
- Smoked salmon with tomato and cream cheese
- Cinnamon breakfast muffins
- 4 ingredient egg casserole
- Tomato, bacon, and melted mozzarella
- Eggs with avocado
- Zucchini frittata

As you can see, eggs play a major part in the breakfast diet here, and that is because they are a) important for health, but also b) very flexible in the Atkins Diet. If you can pack egg of some sort into your breakfast you will have a protein starting point to base the rest of your day on too.

Lunch ideas

Remember that as you go through the day your carb intake is a cumulative effect, so you need to make sure you are using a good carb calculator to keep track. If you try and keep a number in your head and add to it as you go along, you're going to get confused, or make potentially upsetting mistakes which could ruin your phase 1 efforts.

- Chicken and bacon salad
- Asian beef salad
- Egg salad
- Homemade beef burger with feta cheese and tomato
- Buffalo chicken salad
- Cauliflower risotto
- Chicken and ham soup
- Chicken and pesto salad
- Chilli maple mustard ribs
- Tomato and cucumber salad
- Crab and avocado salad
- Cream of mushroom soup
- Guacamole soup
- Creamy chicken and tomato soup

Dinner ideas

- Cheesy cauliflower bake
- Butter chicken
- Cajun fish
- Bacon wrapped cheesy chicken
- Baked meatballs
- Baked Tamari-lemon pork chops
- Sautéed beef with vegetables
- Chicken curry
- Crispy buttermilk fried chicken
- Lamb burgers
- Roast chicken with herbs and lemon
- Jamaican jerk beef

- Pork rind battered fish
- Lamb korma

These dinner ideas are certainly indulgent and don't take up much of your carb intake. Obviously you need to check what you ate at breakfast, lunch, and for your snacks, but provided you don't go over 20g at this stage, you're good to go.

A Few Snack Ideas

Obviously you are going to want to snack a little throughout the day, and it is recommended that if you feel a little hungry between meals, you certainly indulge in a snack or two, provided they fit in with your carb intake allowance.

Here are a few ideas of snacks you might like to try.

- Celery sticks and sour cream or blue cheese
- Cold meats, e.g. ham or turkey
- Pepperoni sticks
- Prawns and dip
- Boiled eggs
- Avocado
- Tuna
- Peanut butter (unsweetened)
- Olives and cheddar cheese
- Cinnamon churritos
- Ham and cheese roll ups
- Scotch eggs
- Vanilla coffee frappe

Most of your favorite foods can be adapted to be Atkins friendly, you simply need to find alternatives to the ingredients that you can't have, such as bread, and then count up the carbs to be sure. This is a great news, because it means that you're never going to feel like you're missing out, provided you simply think outside of the box, count it all up just to be sure (especially during this first phase of the diet), and enjoy in moderation.

Sample Meal Plans

Okay, so let's show you how easy this can be. Here are two weeks of sample meal plans to get you started. You'll see straight away that every day is varied and delicious, totally avoiding the usual boredom factor of a diet – you're not eating anything twice here!

Day 1

Breakfast	-	Turkey sausage sauté with red and green peppers
Lunch	-	Egg salad
Dinner	-	Baked meatballs

Day 2

Breakfast	-	Baked eggs with cheese
Lunch	-	Chicken and bacon salad
Dinner	-	Lamb burgers

Day 3

Breakfast	-	Cinnamon breakfast muffins
Lunch	-	Homemade beef burger with feta cheese and tomato
Dinner	-	Butter chicken

Day 4

Breakfast	-	Zucchini frittata

| Lunch | - | Buffalo chicken salad |
| Dinner | - | Jamaican jerk beef |

Day 5

Breakfast		Smoked salmon with tomato and cream cheese
Lunch	-	Chicken and ham soup
Dinner	-	Beef Chili Stroganoff

Day 6

Breakfast	-	Stuffed Portobello mushrooms
Lunch	-	Chilli maple mustard ribs
Dinner	-	Cajun fish

Day 7

Breakfast	-	4 ingredient egg casserole
Lunch	-	Crab and avocado salad
Dinner	-	Chicken curry

Day 8

Breakfast	-	Mexican breakfast peppers
Lunch	-	Cream of mushroom soup
Dinner	-	Crispy buttermilk fried chicken

Day 9

Breakfast	-	Corned beef hash
Lunch	-	Creamy chicken and tomato soup
Dinner	-	Pork rind battered fish

Day 10

| Breakfast | - | Scrambled eggs with spinach |
| Lunch | - | Asian beef salad |

Dinner   -   Lamb korma

Day 11

Breakfast	-	Tomato, bacon and melted mozzarella
Lunch	-	Cauliflower risotto
Dinner	-	Roasted chicken with herbs and lemon

Day 12

Breakfast	-	Cheese omelet with onions and mushrooms
Lunch	-	Tomato and cucumber salad
Dinner	-	Sautéed beef with vegetables

Day 13

Breakfast	-	Buttermilk cinnamon waffles
Lunch	-	Guacamole soup
Dinner	-	Bacon wrapped cheesy chicken

Day 14

Breakfast	-	Eggs with avocado
Lunch	-	Chicken and pesto salad
Dinner	-	Baked Tamari-lemon pork chops

Points to Remember:

- Always make sure you are getting your correct amount of protein for your weight. Check against current guidelines and make sure you tick that box. Obviously as your weight goes down, your protein allowance will also reduce, but this is a slow process that you should stick to the rules with.
- Never go over 20g of carbohydrates at this point of the diet. You are of course in the first two weeks, and that means you are in phase 1, the most restrictive part of the diet. Having said the word 'restrictive' however, you

should also check the recipes above to see that you can eat some delicious food, without having to worry too much!
- Try and vary your diet as much as possible, by eating different foods every day; this will help you avoid becoming bored, and as a result you will enjoy your diet much more!
- Phase 1 is generally for two weeks at first, but if you want to speed up your weight loss, perhaps if you have more to lose, then it is okay to stay on this phase for longer. As we talked about before, the Atkins Diet is a totally individual deal, and as long as what you are doing is safe and healthy, it is up to you how long you stay on each phase.

The point of this chapter is to give you ideas, to help you see that the Atkins Diet is about much more than being hungry – you won't be hungry! The meal ideas you can see above mean that you can literally eat until you are full, and provided you don't go over that magic 20g of carb figure, there's no reason to stop until you really are satisfied and sated.

There are obviously countless websites and recipe books out there on the market that will show you different recipes to try with the foods you are allowed on the Atkins Diet, and it is a good idea to sit down and have a check of the internet one evening, to give yourself a few ideas. If you can, and you have the time, it's always best to try and plan your meals for the week.

The Advantages of Meal Planning

Obviously there is some room for wiggle here, you don't have to rigidly stick to what you have planned for the week, but if you can try and stick to it as much as possible, you'll save yourself stress and time.

Planning your meals means that:

- You don't have to go shopping every evening after work, when you're hungry and more likely to make rash food decisions
- Don't one large shop at the beginning of the week saves you cash
- You will save time trying to figure out what to eat every single day, which can also lead to unhealthy choices, especially if you leave it too late to decide and you're past the point of hunger
- You can be more creative with your meal planning, giving you more time to think about what you really want
- Spending time working out your meals means that you are more likely to get your protein level correct, as well as sticking to the 20g carb limit during this phase of the diet
- If you are in a household with several other people, and the others aren't following the same diet as you, planning out your meals eliminates confusion

The best advice is to sit down on a Sunday evening, after you have eaten and you're not hungry, and draw out a table for the week – remember, you need breakfast, lunch, dinner, and two snacks per day. Check online for any ideas you might need to come up with, vary your meals, and work it out as you go along, using your carb calculator to make sure the numbers all add up before moving onto the next day. Once you have a full week planned out, write yourself a shopping list of what you need, so you can head to the shops the next day and tick it all off.

Of course, the old adage is certainly true – never go shopping when you're hungry!

The Importance of Exercise

Exercise and the Atkins Diet are not partners that *have* to go together, but it is certainly advantageous for your social life, your appearance, and your health, that you indulge in some exercise at least three times per week. You don't have to head to the gym if you don't want to, but that could be a good way to meet new, likeminded people perhaps. Think about joining exercises classes, such as Zumba, yoga, pilates, step aerobics, kickboxing, spinning – basically anything which you like the sound of. If you can enlist the help of a friend to go with you, all the better!

Obviously during the first phase of the Atkins Diet you can't drink alcohol, because of the high sugar and carb count of alcoholic beverages, and this means that your social life might take a bit of a hit. The key here is to think outside the box and simply alter the way your social life runs – incorporating exercise into it is the ideal way to combine socializing and exercise too.

Exercise is great for your health, which we know, and that is because:

- Exercise reduces the risk of heart disease and stroke

- Blood pressure is lowered, avoiding hypertension (high blood pressure) issues
- You are at less risk of developing diabetes
- Regular exercise (combined with a healthy diet) avoids obesity
- Exercising regularly helps boost your overall energy levels
- You will sleep much better after exercising
- Exercise could give you a social outlet
- Regularly exercising has been shown to improve mood and focus
- Self-confidence and body image is boosted as you see the results of your exercise

If you have a lot of weight to lose, you may find that as you go along you will have excess skin or 'flabby' muscle which needs toning up – exercise can help you with this if you take part in regular activities during the diet you are following; basically, you're toning up as you go along, which gives you much better results in the end.

So, now we know how to do the diet, we know what we can and can't eat, we have a few ideas of delicious foods to try, we know that planning meals is a good idea, and exercise is a wonderful thing, but there is one area of following any diet that you might not be aware of, and something we will discuss in our next chapter.

Read on to reveal all!

Chapter 7:
The Emotional Side of Your Weight Loss Journey

We're going to go a little off-kilter for this chapter, but it's important we show you a well-rounded picture of the journey you're about to go on.

Losing weight isn't just about looking in the mirror and thinking 'wow', whilst loving what you see; of course, that's a big part of it, but there's a much deeper side to weight loss too.

I'm going to talk in this particular chapter on a personal note. Throughout this book we have talked in the 'we' voice, and that is because, well, we're all in it together, right? But, for this particular chapter I want to talk to you person to person, because this is something that is really quite personal too.

I'm going to let you into a little secret, something I learned throughout my own weight loss battle.

Losing weight and maintaining your loss is quite emotional; you will learn quite a lot about yourself and the people around you, you will develop strength and determination you never knew you had in you, and you will end your journey (if it ever really ends) feel extremely proud of yourself, and rightly so.

Let me tell you my story.

I lost around 38kg in weight. I was a big girl, I'll admit, and for a long time I knew it, but I didn't really do anything about it because it was such a huge mountain to climb that I just thought it was impossible. I wasn't at all happy with the way I looked, but to be honest, I loved my food, and I didn't want to give it up!

One particular day I was asked to be a bridesmaid for my friend's wedding, and at first I was really happy about it, that is until the first dress fitting came around. The other bridesmaids were what can only be described as a hell of a lot slimmer than me, and whilst nobody really said anything, I could feel the burning eyes of judgment coming my way. Then came the wedding – I saw the photos, I did not like what the photos showed me, even with several glasses of vodka and alcohol glasses on – something had to change.

Something snapped inside me and I became super focused. I'm not going to lie and tell you it was easy because it wasn't; I had several false starts, I fell off the wagon a few times, and I wondered what on earth I was putting myself through more times than I can remember.

Then I discovered the Atkins Diet.

No, this is not an advert before you wonder, this is actually the truth.

Call me a testimonial for the Atkins Diet if you want to, but the bottom line is that it worked for me and it changed the way I looked at myself. Before trying the Atkins, I was using the old low calorie diet routine, and believe me, I was not a nice person – I was hungry, my god, was I hungry! I often went to bed on an empty stomach, simply to stop myself from raiding the fridge, and I tossed and turned for much of the night, listening to my stomach growl.

Tell me, how is that healthy?

Anyway, the Atkins Diet changed it all, and I found the weight falling off me as I moved my way through the phases, quite happily truth be told. Now, the biggest change began to come my way shortly after my biggest dress size change, and that was that I realized people were treating me differently.

At first I thought this was wonderful – that guy who I had always liked, he suddenly knew I existed! Those girls who never spoke to me before, basically because they were a bit too cool, all of a suddenly they were smiling at me and asking me where I'd bought my dress from.

Can you see where I'm coming from?

Ladies and gentlemen, you will learn that as human beings we are extremely shallow, and that is a rather hard pill to swallow at first. You are the same person inside that you were before you lost your weight, and you'll be the same person inside when you finish your journey – the only difference is that you are smaller than you used to be, and you are healthier too. Is your personality the same? Yes! Do you still believe in the same things? Yes! Is your name the same as it was before? Unless you got married, yes!

Weight loss taught me how vain and shallow human beings are, myself included.

Now, once you make peace with that fact, you get over it and you start to go clothes shopping again, smiling and all happy, but don't ever let yourself forget the lesson it taught you.

When once upon a time I may have been guilty of making the odd joke about someone's size, I now congratulate them on being so confident in their own skin; when I may have judged someone for their actions, something I didn't agree with, I now look a little deeper and accept that everyone has their own path. Basically, weight loss has made me more open minded, less judgmental, and it has made me a more positive person too. Losing weight isn't just about your size, it's about your life, because it alters so much about the way you think, and the way you see the world.

This isn't mumbo-jumbo by the way, I guarantee that you will be thinking the same kinds of things when you reach your goal too.

Confidence is everything, that is something else I have learned.

I wasn't a very confident person when I was at my biggest, in fact I just wanted to hide away and live by myself without scrutiny, but as soon as I began to feel better about myself, my confidence soared. As an example, when I was larger, I was an extremely shy girl, I wouldn't have spoken to anyone first, I certainly wouldn't have gone out of my comfort zone, and I never took risks.

Guess where I am now?

You'll probably never guess, so I'll save you the time.

I'm now living in a foreign country, having moved here on my own and forged my own life, working as a writer, doing the job I always dreamed of, and I have the love of a wonderful man by my side, someone who doesn't care what size I am, or am not. I have even been known to don a bikini during the summer months too, and believe me, that is certainly something that I would never have done a few years ago - body confidence is extremely powerful.

Dreams really can come true, but it's not about magic or luck, it's about confidence and the way you think. You have picked a diet which is much more do-able than many of the others that came before it, and that is means you have a much better shot at succeeding. You only have to read the testimonials to this diet on the Internet to see just how many people have tried and happily reached their targets, and the sheer popularity of it should tell you all you need to know too.

My weight loss journey was very emotional, and yours will be too, but the bottom line of this rather personal out-pouring of mine is to show you one very important thing – when the going gets tough, and no matter how easy the Atkins Diet is, it will get a little tough at some point, whatever you do, don't give up!

Conclusion – Let's Sum It All Up!

So, our journey together is complete!

Hopefully this book will have given you the inspiration, excitement, and positive attitude you need to embark on your own personal weight loss journey. This really is probably going to be the best thing you ever do with your life, because not only are you affecting the way you see yourself, your overall confidence, body confidence, and your dress size, but you're also giving yourself a massive health boost too, which is the most important thing of all.

The most important thing to remember about the Atkins Diet is that it is never really over; once you have reached your weight goal, you need to think about maintenance, and maintenance is simply a different way of saying, 'this is the way I'm going to eat for the rest of my life'.

There is nothing particularly complicated about the Atkins Diet per se, not once you totally understand it, and that is what this book has aimed to help you do. If you can understand something, you know much more about it, and you can follow it with ease, without the worry of falling off the wagon, or making costly mistakes. If you find you're not 100% sure about something, simply head back and re-read over that chapter until you're clear to continue. This book is designed to help you really understand the mechanics of the diet, so you know what is happening to your body through every single phase.

So, to go over it once more – why should you start planning your first Atkins stage right now?

- Fast and guaranteed weight loss
- You will understand your body so much more once you fully understand the diet
- You will learn your carbohydrate tolerance level, which will allow you to maintain your weight loss for life
- The knowledge and power you will receive from learning about food nutrition will arm you with everything you need to live a much healthier and positive life
- Soaring confidence levels as a result of your dramatic loss
- The tools you need to control your weight in the future, knowing exactly what you need to do if you find any weight creeping back on
- You will certainly be needing to buy a new wardrobe, and there is nothing wrong with that!
- You will join a community of other Atkins Dieters, all of whom are extremely supportive and knowledgeable
- Your dietary options will be opened up, as you learn more about what you are eating, and how you can combine different foods for delicious outcomes
- You are the one in control throughout the entire diet

Low carb diets, such as the Atkins Diet, have been proven to give endless health benefits, as well as the number one reason that everyone starts – weight loss fast and dramatically. Nobody wants to endure a diet only to see no result on the scales, and with the Atkins Diet, you certainly don't have that issue to deal with!

Now, we must bid you goodbye, and the only thing left to say is this – good luck!

Eat until you're full, and lose weight?

Welcome to the Atkins Diet!

Check Out My New Book with Delicious Low Carb Recipes!

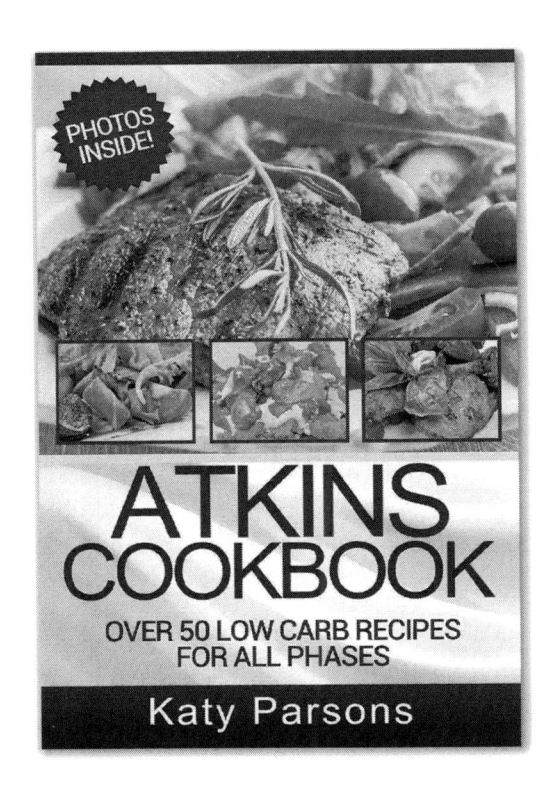

About The Author

Having undergone her own rigorous weight loss battle, Katy Parsons is one of the most sympathetic and real health and diet writers. With an in-depth knowledge of the Atkins Diet and all its major plus points, Katy has helped numerous individuals with her own experiences and information learnt along the way. With the mindset that everyone deserves to feel happy and comfortable in their own skin, no matter what their end goal, Katy stresses the importance of overall health and the lifestyle changes that the Atkins Diet brings in the long-term.

Katy, originally from Boston, currently resides in New York with her husband, three beautiful children, and her precious pet cat. She enjoys traveling as much as possible, creative writing, and rustling up new and delicious recipes to try as part of her own low carb, Atkins Diet lifestyle.

Printed in Great Britain
by Amazon